CONTAGION OF THE NEW MILLENNIUM

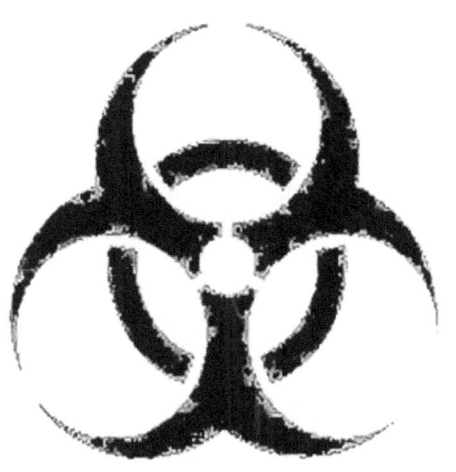

H5N1

SURVIVING THE AVIAN FLU VIRUS

Contagion of the New Millennium
H5N1 - Surviving the Avian Flu Virus

www.createspace.com
7290 B. Investment Drive
Charleston, SC 29418
USA

ISBN-13: 978-1466322851
ISBN-10: 1466322853

Printed in the United States of America

Introduction

To some I suppose this book might be construed as just another conspiracy theory or scare tactic, so to speak. Possibly the scribbling of a slightly neurotic doomsday-sayer similar to your local mentally disturbed vagrant on the street who wears a sign that says "The End is Coming!" I must admit that prior to studying the H5N1 bird flu virus and the potentially devastating effects that it may bring on society and civilization as a whole; I too was somewhat skeptical and indifferent on the subject. To think that something as minute and insignificant as a simple contagion such as a flu virus, could cripple our country, destroy our economy and kill one out of every two people who become infected with it almost seem ludicrous; like a bad episode of The Twilight Zone. Not something which could ever occur now at the dawn of the 21st century; a time of sophisticated robotics, multi-processor PC's, alternate energy vehicles, artificial hearts, shopping malls and MP3 players. A time when man can travel beyond the moon, probe neighboring planets and harness the power of the atom. The thought that an obscure microscopic organism which primarily infects birds half way around the world could influence us or impact our lives in the least, let alone kill us and our loved ones; all seemed pretty preposterous at best. It wasn't until I did my own research about this particular virus that I drew the conclusion that this is going to be a really major event which could potentially change the world as we know it. Borders, governments, economies, ecosystems, institutions, utilities, regulations, routines, allies, enemies, threats, safe havens, family structure, relationships, etc., once this pandemic event begins, no one will be safe from its ensuing destruction and the chaotic madness soon to follow in its wake. The only ones who will be capable of surviving will be those who have prepared in advance for the upcoming disastrous events. Those who have taken steps well in advance to protect themselves, their loved ones and family members prior to the invasion of this deadly strain. Hopefully everyone who reads this book will find the information both informative and useful in planning, evading and surviving this modern day plague.

A Word of Caution

Many of the topics and events which are discussed in this book may be disturbing to some readers. It is not the intent of the author to create a state of fear, but rather to notify the general public of a potentially hazardous threat to society. This publication was written and intended for informative purposes only. All of the contents within this book are believed to be true; however, the author makes no claims as to the accuracy and validity of its contents and will not be held liable for any loss of life, limb, property, economic, mental, social or emotional faculties and/or functions which may be negatively affected, influenced, diminished and/or altered in anyway as a result of the use and/or implementation of any of the mentioned topics, events, products and/or techniques proposed and/or suggested herein.

Special Thanks

Special thanks to of my incredibly talented and knowledgeable friends for helping me with the tedious research and endless fact-finding tasks that were involved with the writing of this book. Their continuous assistance and editing skills helped make this book possible.

Table of Contents

Chapter 1
What is the H5N1 Virus

H5N1 is also known as a subtype of the Influenza A virus, or A(H5N1). A bird-adapted strain called HPAI A(H5N1) for "Highly Pathogenic Avian Influenza virus of type A of subtype H5N1", is the causative agent of H5N1 flu, commonly known as "Avian Influenza" or "Bird Flu". This particular virus has been affecting many bird populations in Southeast Asia and one strain is spreading globally, killing tens of millions of birds. The first known strain of HPAI A(H5N1) killed two flocks of chickens in Scotland in 1959; however, that strain was very different from the current highly pathogenic strain we have today. Infected birds transmit H5N1 through their saliva, nasal secretions, feces and blood. Other animals may become infected with the virus through direct contact with these bodily fluids or through contact with surfaces contaminated with them.

The virus can also remain infectious after 30 days at 32.0°F (freezing temperatures) or 6 days at 98.6°F (human body temperatures). In frigid Arctic temperatures, it does not degrade at all. There is currently no evidence of efficient human-to-human transmission or of airborne transmission of HPAI A(H5N1) to humans. In almost all cases examined, those infected with H5N1 had extensive physical contact with infected birds. Still, approximately 60% of humans known to have been infected with the Asian strain of HPAI A(H5N1) have died from it. That's a mortality rate of over fifty percent! The H5N1 is thought by top virologists to be on the verge of mutating into a strain which will become highly contagious to humans and spread easily via coughing, sneezing and direct physical contact.

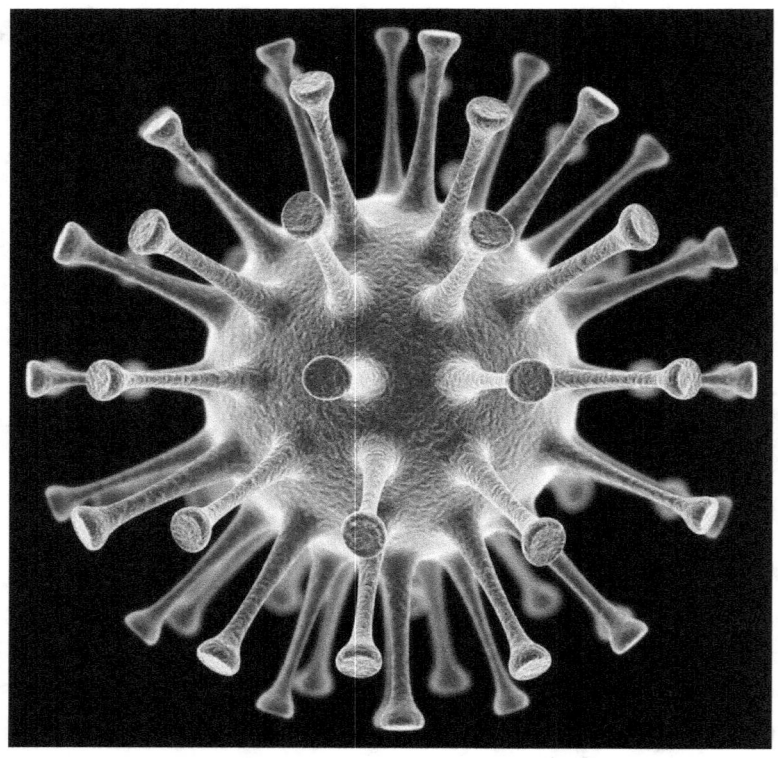

Influenza Virus as Seen Under an Electron Microscope

Here are just a few other documented viruses from the past, and a brief description of the impact they had:

H1N1
This virus caused the "Spanish flu" also known as the 1918 flu pandemic. It lasted from 1918 to 1919 and caused an estimated 660,000 deaths in the US and an estimated 50 to 100 million worldwide. This strain currently causes seasonal human flu, and caused the 2009 flu pandemic known as the "Swine flu".

H2N2

This virus caused the "Asian flu" which originated in China and lasted from 1956 to 1958. It was the result of a viral mutation from wild ducks combined with a pre-existing human strain. The death toll in the US alone was around 70,000 with an infection rate of 1 to 4 million.

H3N2

This virus caused the "Hong Kong flu" which lasted from 1968 to 1969. It was a descendant strain of the H2N2. In the US there were over 50 million people infected with roughly 34,000 deaths. This strain currently causes seasonal human flu.

Viruses of lesser severity include the following:

H1N2

First Reported in 1988, currently endemic in humans and pigs and causes seasonal human flu

H9N2

First Reported in 1999, known to have infected three people

H7N7

First Reported in 2003, unusual potential for species transfer, known to have killed one person

H7N2

First Reported in 2002, known to have infected two people

H7N3

First Reported in 1979, known to have infected two people

H10N7

First Reported in 1979, known to have infected two people

Chapter 2
Bird Flu vs. Traditional Strains

When people think of the flu, the symptoms which typically come to mind are fever, chills, headache, sneezing, runny nose, sore throat, muscle aches, fatigue, etc. When flu season comes around we are warned to take precautions against whatever the latest strain is that is coming out of Asia that year, and urged to get a flu vaccine from our family doctor. Usually this warning is directed primarily toward children, the elderly, and those with weakened immune systems. Historically various flu strains tend to hit hardest and result in the highest amount of death on this segment of the population. However, for the majority of us who are in a healthy state prior to acquiring the latest "bug" going around the office, lodge, church or weekly social gathering, getting the flu is nothing more than a minor annoyance or interruption in our lives which will disrupt a few days of our daily routines while we curl up with a warm blanket, TV, chicken noodle soup and some type of over the counter cold and flu relief medicine.

Unfortunately, when you mention the bird flu to someone in America, this is probably the same thoughts that they conjure up in their minds. Mention H5N1 and you might as well be speaking in binary. With over 1,400 infectious diseases floating around, most people do not have a clue what the differences are between a common flu and the H5N1 bird flu, and many just do not care. This benign view and trivialization of the virus is what may ultimately cause the unnecessary deaths of countless millions of people, both here and abroad. With H5N1, a person can not only be infected, but also be contagious for two days or more before showing signs or symptoms of the virus. Once symptoms do develop, they will hit hard and overwhelm the immune system. If fact, those below the age of 43, who have a quicker responding immune system, will be at risk the most. This is primarily due to the body's defense system producing something called cytokine at the first onset of infection. When the response fails to neutralize the virus, the body simply continues to produce greater amounts of the pro-inflammatory to the point that they reach toxic levels within the body. The results are that the inner lining of the lungs begin to break down, ooze and bleed. The lungs are overwhelmed with the fluids produced. Ultimately the person will end up drowning in their own blood and fluids. Upon the onset of these symptoms, the victim would most certainly need to be hospitalized and placed on a respiratory ventilator to have any chance of survival. Even then there's a 60% chance that they won't pull through. Right now there are no vaccines for the H5N1 bird flu virus. The only medications which are thought to be of some use combating the disease are antiviral drugs such as Tamiflu® (oseltamivir) or Relenza® (zanamivir). At one point the US government took these drugs off the shelves in order to stock pile them for use by governmental agencies and first responders. At present Canada has enough Tamiflu® for 17% of their population, France enough for 20%, England enough for 25% and the US enough for 1%. It is still not known just how effective today's antiviral drugs will be at combating the H5N1 virus. The use of antiviral medications will only halt the advancement of the disease and not create any long term immunities to the virus. Actual vaccines against the virus cannot be produced until the first human-to-human cases occur from the mutated strain. Once a sample has been obtained from an infected pandemic victim, it would have to be sent to special labs where scientists would work to disarm the virus by genetically altering it so that commercial manufacturers could safely mass produce vaccine. This process would take roughly 2 months. Once commercial manufacturers received the modified virus it would take another 3 to 4 months before the first synthesized vaccines could start to be shipped out. This means that everyone would be open to infection for half a year prior to any vaccines even becoming available. The first batches that are produced would only be enough to cover approximately 9% of the global population. It would take a few more months to produce the millions of additional doses needed to supply people worldwide. Most would say "So what. Six months to a year is nothing. After all, how fast can a simple flu virus spread anyway?" To put this into prospective, we could examine what happened during the first wave of the 1918 virus H1N1. This wave ran from approximately September 14th to October 5th of that same year, in which time the H1N1 virus was able to spread across the country, from New York City to California, from Florida to Washington State; and that was back in 1918. Imagine how much the world has changed

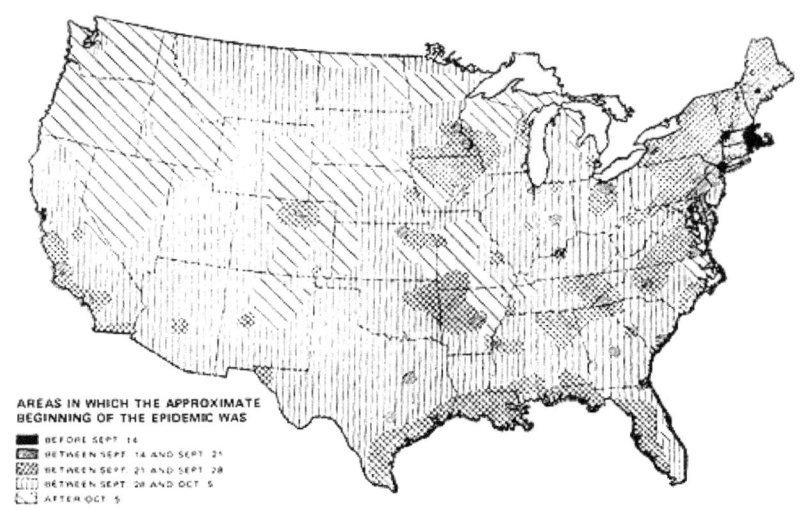

AREAS IN WHICH THE APPROXIMATE
BEGINNING OF THE EPIDEMIC WAS

- BEFORE SEPT 14
- BETWEEN SEPT 14 AND SEPT 21
- BETWEEN SEPT 21 AND SEPT 28
- BETWEEN SEPT 28 AND OCT 5
- AFTER OCT 5

Chart Showing the First Wave of the Virus of 1918

today with all the improvements in the transportation industry (i.e. - airplanes, buses, subways, trains, car rentals, etc.). All of these represent excellent methods for a cross-state, cross-country and cross-continental distribution of the H5N1 virus to easily occur in a matter of a few short hours. The Los Alamos National Laboratory in New Mexico ran a computer simulation of the spread of the H5N1 virus in the US and found that the virus would spread to virtually every town and city in America within three months. Just think of all the publicly exposed or exchanged items that most of us come in contact with everyday such as: door knobs, handrails, keypads on ATM's, credit cards, coins and cash, buttons on a copy machine, public telephones, video rentals, the keyboard or mouse of a computer, nozzles on gas pumps, food trays at fast food restaurants, handles on shopping carts, toilet seats, hotel rooms, amusement parks and rides, shared food or drinks between family members or loved ones, even a simple kiss good-bye. The potential modes for spreading and contracting the virus are endless. If fact, it's predicted that during the pandemic, the number of new infections and deaths would double every 3 days.

The US Secretary of Health & Human Services, Mike Leavitt, is quoted as saying that he thought it was virtually inevitable that a pandemic would occur.

World Health Organization (WHO) estimates that up to 500,000 people are traveling on planes at any one time. This not only has the potential for creating a forced breeding ground for airborne viruses contained within air-tight fuselages housing hundreds of people at a time, but also transferring a highly infectious contagion all around the world at 600mph, 24/7. Just think of all the people that could come in physical contact with just one infected passenger. Let's go through a simple scenario. Presume we follow an infected passenger's travel throughout his trip for just one day and see how many objects he contaminates and people he inadvertently infects. Let's say the passenger is going on a business trip to meet with a few clients. He was infected the

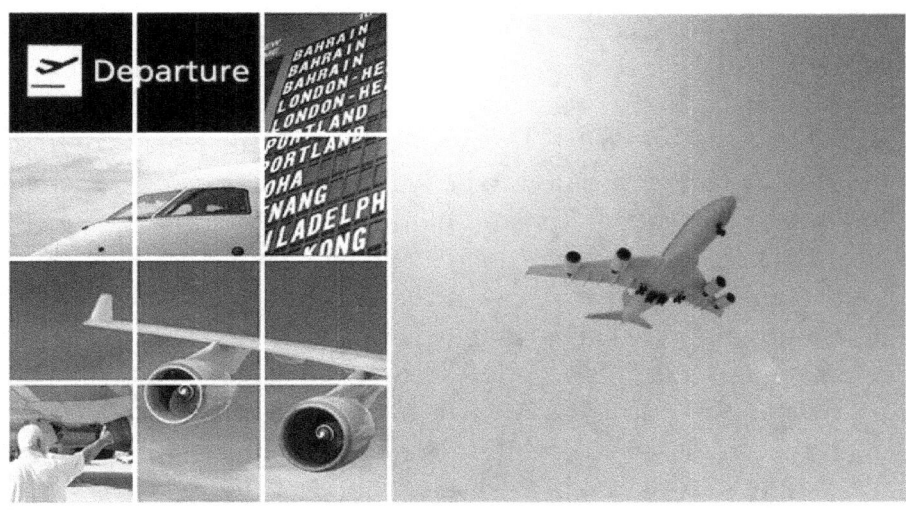

Jetliners Bound for Destinations Across the Globe

night before while eating out at a local restaurant. He wakes with a minor runny nose and a slight cough, causing him to periodically wipe his nose and cough into his hand. He packs his bags and calls a taxi to pick him up from his home. As he waits by the sidewalk, his neighbor jogs by. They high five each other, chat for a moment then part company. *Now his neighbor is infected.* The taxi arrives and the passenger opens the back door using the outside handle, then closes the door using the inside handle. *Now both handles are contaminated.* He sits in the taxi for a half hour plus, touching the seats and arm rest. *Now the back area of the taxi is contaminated.* He arrives at the airport and counts up the fair which he hands to the taxi driver. *Now the taxi driver is infected.* A skycap helps the passenger with his luggage into the airport, holding it by the same handles that the infected passenger was holding 30 seconds prior. *Now the skycap is infected.* The passenger goes into the airport and stands in line at the ticket counter, brushing against others who are also waiting, and holding onto the railing. *Now the railing is contaminated and some of the people waiting are infected.* He checks his bag and hands the ticketing agent his papers, identification, and leans over onto the counter. *Now the ticketing agent is infected and the counter is contaminated.* He uses the pen at the counter to sign his signature. *Now the pen is contaminated.* He makes his way to the security line where again he waits in line, brushing against others also waiting in line and holding onto the railing. *Again more railing is contaminated and more people waiting in the security line are infected.* At security he has to put his personal items into a bin for the x-ray machine. *Now the bin is contaminated.* He gets through security and makes his way to his concourse. Along the way he stops by a vendor for a cup of coffee and a newspaper. He browses through a few magazines before making his selection. *Now the magazines are contaminated.* He counts out the cash and hands it to the vendor. *Now the vendor is infected.* He gets to his terminal and sits down in a chair to wait while he drinks his coffee and reads his newspaper. When the plane begins to board he pushes up off the chair with his hands. *Now the chair is contaminated.* He leaves the newspaper on the nearby table for someone else to read. *Now the newspaper is contaminated.* As he goes toward the gate, he pushes open a trash bin door to throw his empty coffee cup away. *Now the trash bin door is contaminated.* He boards the plane and hands his boarding pass to the attendant who points him to his seat location. *Now the attendant is infected.* Before he gets to his seat, he helps someone stow their bag in an overhead compartment. *Now their bag is contaminated.* He continues to his seat, touching head and arm rests along the way to steady himself. *Now those head and arm rests are contaminated.* He sits down continues to contaminate his immediate surroundings and everything he touches or comes in contact with, including the passengers he was sitting next to. He sneezes a few times and coughs throughout the flight. *Now a majority of the other passengers in the plane are infected.* He arrives at his destination, deplanes and proceeds to baggage claim. In the meantime, several luggage handlers have loaded and unloaded his bags

at the departure and arrival airports. *Now they are infected.*
Along the way to baggage claim, he stops by the restroom. He
opens a stall and locks it from the inside. *Now the door handles
on the stall are contaminated.* He flushes the toilet and uses the
sink. *Now the handles on the sink and toilet are contaminated.* He
gets to baggage claim and decides to get a cart for his luggage.
Now the luggage cart is contaminated. After getting his luggage,
he leaves the airport via another taxi. *Again the door handles
and inside of the taxi are contaminated.* He pays the driver.
Again another driver is infected. After checking into his hotel
where he continues to contaminate countless items and areas,
and infect hotel guests and staff, he proceeds to his business
meeting where he shakes hands with a two dozen people.
Now those people are infected. The next day he heads back home
and repeats the same level of contaminating and infecting all
over again. Just imagine for a moment the number of people
that would be infected and spread the contagion in any given
day, just from that first taxi ride. When you start to look at all
of the people who were infected, as well as the objects and
locations that were contaminated in our little scenario, it's
fairly easy to see how a virus outbreak could turn into a full
blown pandemic so quickly, especially in our modern day
society.

Chapter 3
Advanced Preparation

The first things to look at when attempting advanced preparation for a cataclysmic event such as the bird flu pandemic is what you will need to survive, physically, mentally and emotionally. One good place to start might be to take a look at Maslow's Hierarchy of Needs. This is a theoretical model in psychology that Abraham Maslow proposed in his 1945 paper *A Theory of Human Motivation*. It shows man's most basic needs in human life, then builds upon that foundation to include several progressively complex psychological components.

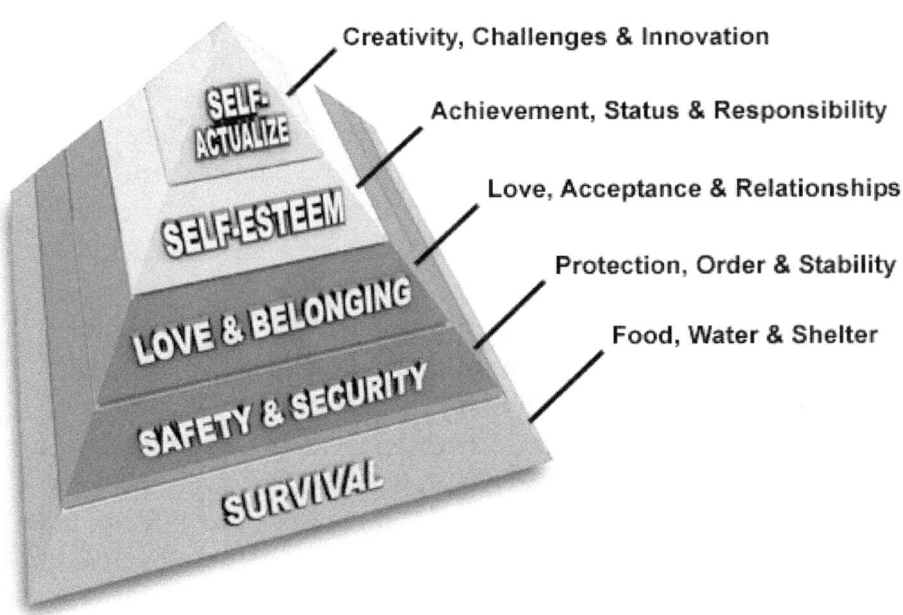

Modified Version of Maslow's Hierarchy of Needs

Although I won't be addressing every level in this pyramid, the base levels of the hierarchy pertains to such things as air, food, water, sleep, safety, security and resources. All are good starting points to examine when it comes to basic survival, so that is where we'll begin.

Air

Clean, purified air is essential to staying healthy and uninfected during a flu pandemic. One of the safest places to avoid any type of airborne contagion would be inside a sealed, underground bunker with a state-of-the-art air purification system. Since this type of complex structure is probably out of the reach of most Americans, your home is probably your next best bet, especially one with a basement. However, even a well sealed house can still be infiltrated by the bird flu. But there are things you can do to improve the air purity cycling through your home. The first is to change out the air filters in your air conditioning/furnace units (HVAC system) for a good electrostatic or allergen type air filter. These types of filters won't necessarily stop a bird flu virus, but they can help to capture and trap many kinds of airborne contaminants and at least in part, help reduce your risks of exposure. You could also look at installing a HEPA (High Efficiency Particulate Air) filtration system in your home. HEPA filters can remove at least 99.97% of airborne particles 0.3 microns in diameter and larger. These systems can be small units that filter the air in individual rooms, or larger systems which attach directly to your home's central air system and clean the air while it circulates through the ductwork. Again, these types of filters may not filter out all bird flu viruses that pass through it, which can range in size from 0.08 to 0.12 microns, but they will help to capture and trap a wide array of other airborne contaminants that viruses may be hitching a ride on, which in turn may further help reduce your risks of exposure.

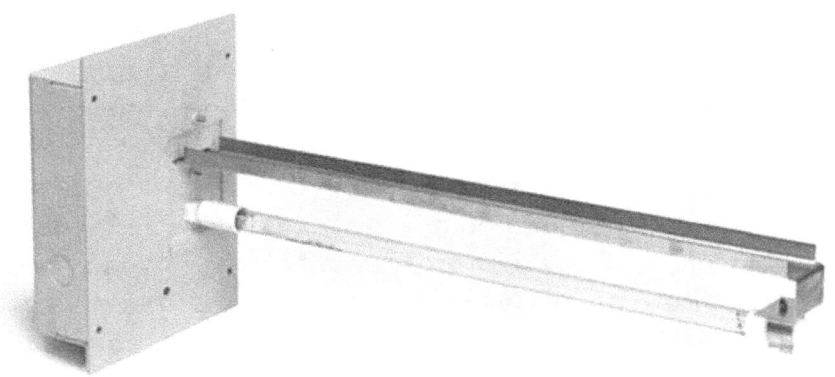

A Typical Germicidal Lamp Used in HVAC Units

Another component to consider in the fight for air purity is what's called a photo-catalytic UV-C air cleaner (germicidal lamp). These are high intensity UV (ultra-violet) tubes which simply insert through a hole cut into the distribution duct of your air conditioning / furnace unit (HVAC system). The light produced by these tubes is similar to that emitted by the sun. The high intensity UV light basically destroys the DNA of viruses that pass by it, essentially making them sterile, assuming they survive. Therefore, if someone later comes in contact with the sterilized virus, and it enters their body, it will be unable to duplicate itself and multiply. So, once that single virus cell dies, it's the end of that virus and the person exposed remains uninfected. One of the best solutions to exposure is all out avoidance of the outside world as much as possible. If you must adventure outdoors for any reason, it will be imperative that you wear a good face mask that has a tight seal and can filter airborne particles down to 0.3 microns or less. Make sure that the masks you use have a rating of N100. The more common N95 masks will give you a false sense of security if you use them against H5N1 or any virus for that matter. They will not offer you enough protection. There is one mask on the market called the NanoMask® which will not only block the H5N1 virus, but chemically kill it as well. It is capable of filtering out bacteria and particles 3 times smaller than the flu virus (see table below). It should be noted that a face mask alone may not stop a virus from infecting you, as other parts of your body may put you at equal risk of exposure, such as your eyes, hands, open sores, etc. Always wear disposable gloves and eye protection as well. If you have any cuts or sores, be sure to cover them with a proper bandage or dressing. Disposable coveralls and shoe covers could go a long way in reducing the level of contamination of your clothes as well. Remember, the H5N1 is a hearty virus which can survive for days on an open surface. Do everything you can to avoid unwarranted exposure.

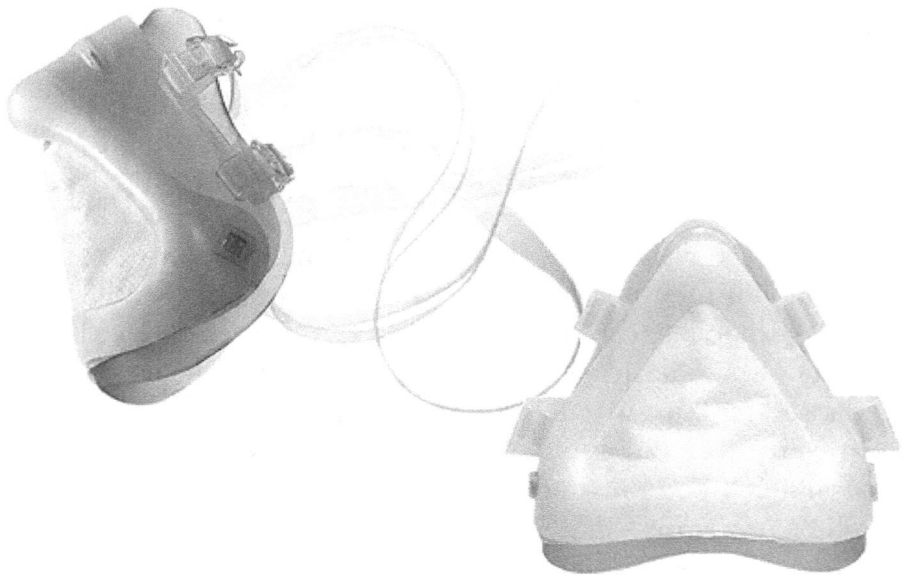

NanoMask® - Manufactured by Emergency Filtration Products

Viruses		
Species	**Size in Microns**	**Associated Dieases**
Bacteriophage ØX174	0.025 to 0.027 diameter	Test virus used by Nelson Laboratories to test 2H Technology™ filtration efficiencies
Hepatitis Virus (HBV)	0.042 to 0.047 diameter	Hepatitis B
Adenovirus	0.07 to 0.09 diameter	Respiratory Infections
HIV	0.08 to 0.11 diameter	Acquired Immunodeficiency Syndrome
Filoviruses	0.08 diameter 0.79 to 0.97 length	Ebola Virus
Bunyaviridae	0.08 to 0.12 diameter	Hanta Virus
Orthomyxoviridae	0.08 to 0.12 diameter	Influenza A, B and C
Coronaviridae (SARS-CoV)	0.10 to 0.12 diameter	SARS
Varicella-Zoster Virus	0.11 to 0.12 diameter	Herpes
Cytomegalovirus	0.12 to 0.20 diameter	Pneumonia, Hepatitis, Retinitis, Encephalitis
Variola Virus	0.14 to 0.26 diameter 0.22 to 0.45 length	Small Pox
Bacteria		
Serratia Marcescens	0.45 diameter	Extraintestinal Infections, Nosocomial Infections
Pseudomonas Aeruginosa	0.50 to 1.0 diameter 1.5 to 4.0 length	Endocarditis, Pneumonia, Osteomyelitis, Nosocomial Infections, Meningitis, Septicemia
Staphylococcus Aureus	1.0 diameter	Pneumonia, Osteomyelitis, Acute Endocartis Meningitis, Toxic Shock Syndrome, Myocarditis
Mycobacteriumtuberculosis	1.0 to 5.0 diameter	Tuberculosis
Bacillus Anthracis	1.0 to 1.5 diameter 3.0 to 5.0 length	Anthrax Infection

Table Showing the Sizes of Various Viral and Bacterial Contaminants

In September of 2001, following the terrorist attacks on the Twin Towers & Pentagon, letters containing weaponized anthrax spores, were mailed to several news media offices and two Democratic US Senators, killing 5 people and infecting 17 others. Soon after, government officials began to advise residents to buy duct tape and plastic sheeting, so they could create a makeshift "safe room" in their homes, where they could seek refuge in the event of a larger scale terroristic attack. The problem which they failed to address was how to supply fresh air to those inside. As this was not mentioned, the presumption is that plastic over windows and duct tape around the gaps of doors is not likely to be "air tight". If that is true, then we must also assume that contaminated air would leak into the safe room as well. Even so, the principle is relatively sound. One solution to addressing this problem would be to install a positive pressure, biological filtration system, with a built-in UV germicidal lamp. This type of system would draw in fresh air from the outside, filter out allergens & contaminates and sanitize any viruses, while creating a positive pressure in the room. This consistent influx of air would make the pressure inside higher than that outside, thus forcing air out of any cracks, gaps or crevasses, ensuring that no viruses or contagions are able to leak in. Usually these systems come with a back-up battery, power generator and/or manual hand pump. This is similar to the type of systems that many hospitals use in their infectious disease wards. If you're wondering how big of a system you might need, figuring out the air consumption requirements for a room is fairly easy once you know how many people may be in it. The average adult in a calm state of rest requires a minimum of 5 cubic feet of fresh air every minute (cfm) to survive. However, when people are panicked or under stress, the demand can be as much as three times that (see table below), so consider this before settling on a system size.

People at Rest			
Room Size	Room Air Volume in Cubic Feet	Number of People	Minimum Air Volume Needed
10'Lx10'Wx7.5'H	750	1	2.5 cfm
10'Lx10'Wx7.5'H	750	2	5.0 cfm
10'Lx10'Wx7.5'H	750	4	10.0 cfm
People Under Stress			
Room Size	Room Air Volume in Cubic Feet	Number of People	Minimum Air Volume Needed
10'Lx10'Wx7.5'H	750	1	5.0 cfm
10'Lx10'Wx7.5'H	750	2	10.0 cfm
10'Lx10'Wx7.5'H	750	4	20.0 cfm

Table of Fresh Air Requirements of Adults at Rest & Under Stress

Food

Undoubtedly food will be one of the most crucial items you must stock up on during your advanced preparations. Not only do you need to be smart about how you store your food, you must also be smart about what type of food you are going to store as well. The most convenient type of foods to store are what people refer to as Meals Ready to Eat (MRE's). MRE's are food rations commonly used by the U.S. military and other various disaster relief organizations or agencies. These shelf stable foods require no cooking or re-hydration and can be eaten hot or cold.

Unlike their predecessors, today's MRE's are packed in flexible pouches that are tough and durable and typically have an average shelf life of 5-10 years depending on storage temperatures and conditions (see Graph 1). MRE's come in a wide selection of meals such as Beef Stroganoff, Beef Stew, BBQ Chicken, Chicken Noodle Stew, Cheese Tortellini, Vegetarian Chili, etc. with a variety of side items and deserts.

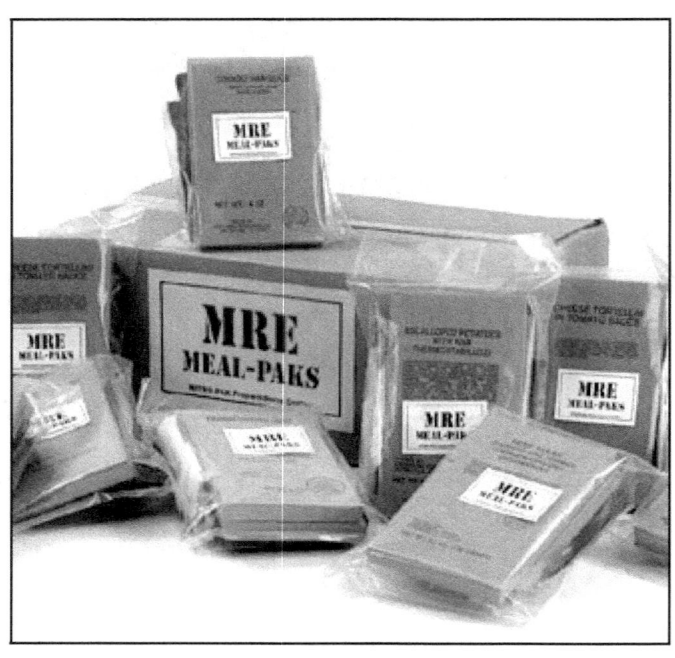

Typical Meals Ready to Eat (MRE's) Packaging

Each MRE has an average of 1,100-1,300 calories, which replicates the calorie count of a complete meal. Sometimes they can have lofty retail pricing, so shop around before you buy. If you're in a hurry and don't want to go through the hassle of manually stocking up on different types of dried & can goods, then MRE's might be for you.

For the rest of you who may want to piece mill your own emergency rations, here is what I recommend. Typically the average adult needs to consume approximately 1,200 calories per day to maintain proper health and bodily functions. When caloric intake falls below 1,200 per day, it becomes difficult to obtain all the nutrients that are needed by the body to stay strong & energetic and prevent diseases. Very low calorie intakes can also lead to other health problems such as gout, gallstones, heart complications, etc., so keep this in mind

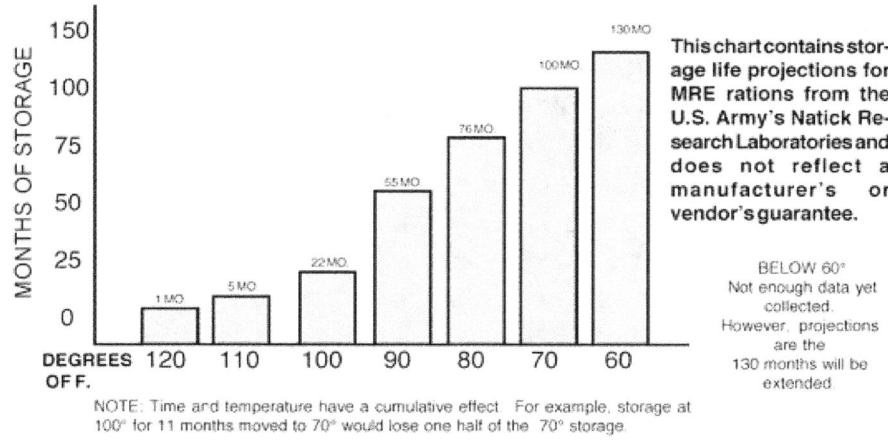

Graph of Shelf Life Projections of MRE's vs. Temperature

when grocery shopping for emergency rations. Buy large cans of vegetables such as corn, beans, peas, spinach, beets and potatoes, any of which can range in cost from $2.50 to $5.00 at your local supermarket. Canned chili with beans and corned beef hash are also high in calories. Rice, dried beans, instant mashed potatoes, and dehydrated noodle soups are also excellent sources of carbohydrates to maintain energy levels. They also tend to have a much higher shelf life than canned goods. Besides, a 50lbs of rice could go a long way, but don't rely on it for much nutritional value. Store up on lots of salt, both powdered and rock. It's cheap and it can be used to preserve other foods later on if necessary. Make sure it's iodized though. Iodized salt is salt which has been fortified with iodine to prevent endemic goiters (enlargement of the thyroid) from forming on the throat. Always look at the expiration dates of whatever it is that you are buying. If it will not last for at least two years or more, consider getting something else. Many times it may be tempting to buy giant jars of pickles or olives since they appear to be healthy snacks and seem to last forever, but resist the urge. The amount of nutritional value for such foods is practically zero. If you ate an entire jar of these types of food items every day, you could still starve to death. Tuna fish, peanut butter, apple sauce and Vienna sausages are also good long-term storage items to look at. In addition, think about storing food prep and condiment items such as cooking oil, vinegar, soy sauce, Worcestershire sauce, powdered gravy mix, sugar, flour, pepper and spices. Eventually if your food supplies do run out, you might need these items to complete or enhance the flavor of food that has been grown or caught, such as fish, wild game or even food which may be supplied by the Red Cross, FEMA, NATO, the UN or some other relief effort.

Figuring out just how much food you are going to need will be dependant on how many people you need to store food for and how long you expect to be isolated. Many experts feel that the bird flu pandemic may impact this country for as long as 6 to 8 months. Based on this I would recommend storing up 6 months worth of supplies, minimum. Don't forget goodies and snacks, maybe even candy or gum, but remember to keep an eye on the expiration dates. Items like cookies and crackers tend to go stale much faster than more durable dried goods.

Water

Aside from air, water is the second most important item needed for basic human survival. The human body is made up of roughly 65% water. This water is needed for circulation and other critical bodily processes including respiration and converting food to energy. To maintain ones health and efficiency, a minimum of two (2) quarts of clean water per day per person is the generally accepted rule of thumb, so plan accordingly when storing water supplies. Powdered orange breakfast drink is a good source of vitamin C which will be necessary to prevent such nutrient deficient diseases such as scurvy which can occur from lack of citrus. So consider stocking up on this type of drink additive. Other items you may want to store are instant coffee, hot chocolate mix, powdered milk, fruit drink mix, etc.

In addition to drinking water, you might want to think about larger storage units for washing and bathing. During a pandemic there is always the risk that basic utilities, such as water treatment plants, may fail due to maintenance issues and/or lack of employees showing up for work.

If water supplies run low for whatever reason, you will want to have a way of filtering various water sources, such as rain water, pond water, water from streams or lakes, etc. To effectively do this you should consider getting some type of water filtration device that is gravity fed, such as one using ceramic filters or better. Even though super filters can filter out as much as 99.9999% of viruses, boiling the water prior to filtration would still be a good idea.

If filtered water is not an option, untreated water can still be sanitized using regular liquid bleach. Use 8 drops per gallon of water, or ½ teaspoon per five gallons. If the water being treated is cloudy, double the amount of bleach used.

Sleep

During a heightened event such as a bird flu pandemic, many people may find it difficult to get rest or sleep while facing so many adverse problems, risks and even their own mortality; yet it is important to get the proper amount of sleep and rest that your body needs, seven (7) – nine (9) hours per day. Lack of sleep can not only make you groggy and unable to function at peak performance if needed, it can disrupt all kinds of physiological functions of the body, not to mention lowering your immune system. The last thing you need during a flu pandemic is to get sick with some other illness that may cause you to have to go to one of the already overstrained hospitals or healthcare facilities. This would almost certainly result in becoming infected with the H5N1 virus. Storing up on some over the counter sleeping aids may prove to be an invaluable move in the long run.

Waste

Let's face it, when we think of food, water and supplies, sanitation and toiletry items are probably the last thing on our minds, yet tackling a small problem such as waste disposal can quickly become an insurmountable problem. Improper sewage disposal can lead to the possibility of contracting other serious diseases or illnesses such as:

- Gastroenteritis, characterized by cramping stomach pains, diarrhea and vomiting.
- Hepatitis, characterized by inflammation of the liver, and jaundice.
- Allergic alveolar (inflammation of the lung) with fever, breathlessness, dry cough, aching muscles and joints.

Furthermore, the H5N1 virus can also be spread by flying insects such as flies and mosquitoes, so attracting such insects with garbage or raw sewage is one of the last things you will want to do. As discussed earlier in this chapter, there is always the risk that basic utilities such as water may fail. If this happens, do not use the toilets in your home or you will run the risk of long term exposure to raw sewage inside your home. To combat this problem, look at getting a portable chemical toilet. One of the advantages to a chemical toilet is the liquid inside which not only acts as a deodorizer, but a disinfectant as well. Chemical toilets can be as simple as a 5 gallon bucket with a snap on toilet seat or as complicated as a deluxe flushable model with a built-in water reservoir. When the time comes to empty these type units, or dispose of trash and garbage, you should be sure to dig a hole nearby and bury it. If you house uses a fresh water well, make sure waste is disposed far enough away as to not contaminate the water

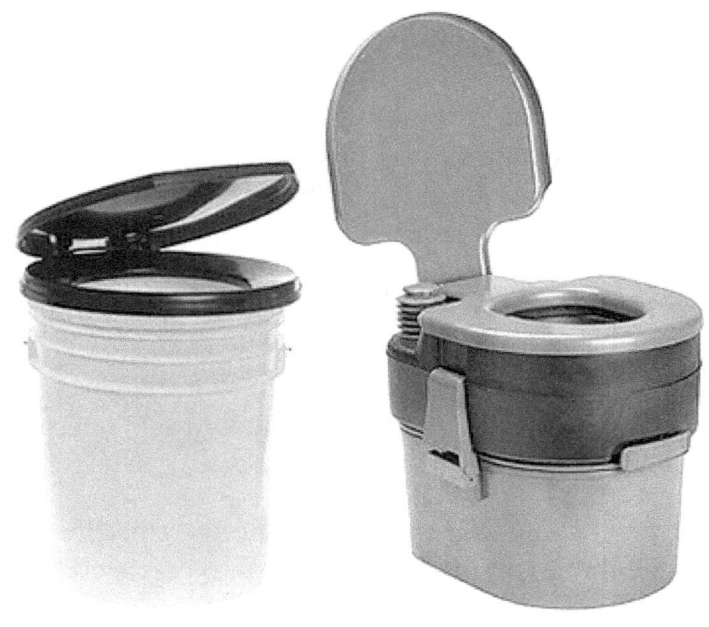

Basic Chemical Toilet (left), Deluxe, Flushable Model (right)

source via runoff or leaching. Either way, emptying a portable toilet or changing out its internal bucket, certainly beats the alternatives. In addition to the toilet, don't forget to stock up on toilet paper. The dumbest thing in the world would be to contract the bird flu because you had to go out and track down some bathroom tissue. Finally, remember disposable cups, plates, eating utensils and napkins too. You won't want to waste precious drinking water washing dirty dishes if you don't have to.

Expendable Items

Besides bathroom tissue, be sure to include other toiletry items to your list which would encompass bathing, shaving, dental hygiene, grooming and feminine products as well. Take a hard look at what you and your family consume every week then plan accordingly.

Security & Safety

When it comes to security, nothing beats a good alarm system. But what if the electricity to your home is off or worse yet, what if the police just are not responding to break-ins anymore. Having a dog for protection might be a good alternative. Dogs often make a great deterrent to someone wanting to break in, because they can not only warn you of a potential intruder, but can defend you as well. They also make great companions and contribute to the social family structure. If you do decide to get a dog, or have one already, don't forget to stock up on dog food as well.

Assume that at some point there may not be electricity for lighting. Stocking-up on flash lights and batteries is a great idea, but if the pandemic lasts for six months or more, will you have enough? Fumbling around in the dark every night would be neither fun nor safe. One solution is flash lights and lanterns which you can recharge by shaking, cranking or

placing in direct sunlight. There are dozens of different models on the market to choose from. Some of these even come with a built-in radio or television as well. Be sure at least one of your units has a radio or TV attached so you can stay informed with current news, events and announcements. Radios that can pick-up short wave are best because, depending on the time of day or night, you would be able to pick-up broadcasts from all around the world.

It may seem a little far fetched to think of fortifying your house against a potential home invasion, but that is exactly one of the items that may ultimately save your life. As resources become scarce and people become more desperate

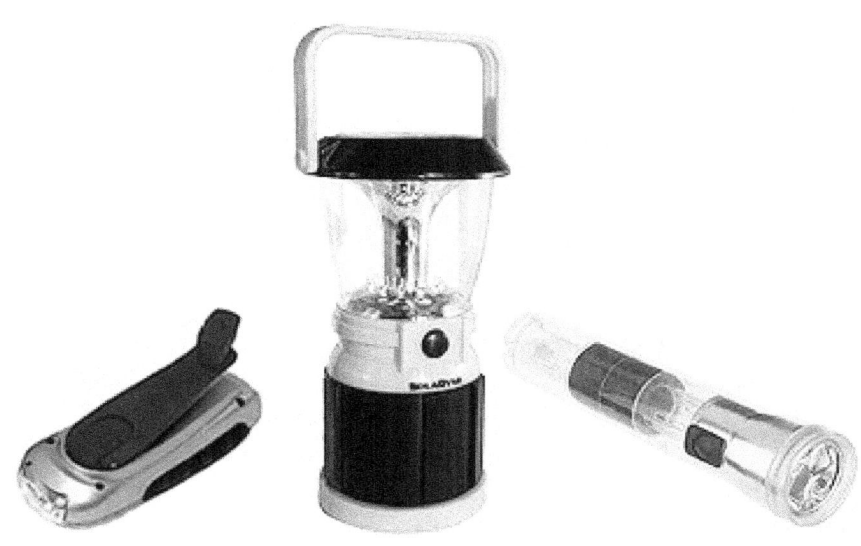

Various Types of Rechargeable Lights on the Market Today

for food and everyday supplies, it's not just conceivable that home invasions will become more common, it's likely. We've all heard the phrase "desperate times call for desperate measures", which precisely describes the rationalization that most people on the street will be thinking as they resort to violence to obtain much needed items from others. You can see this type of behavior in riots or civil unrest, where people seem to revert to primal behavior when together in a hostile crowd. When a few people begin to engage in unlawful behavior, others in the crowd will often cheer and egg them on. This results in escalating violence as others in the crowd begin to believe that the anonymity of the crowd and the safety in numbers will protect them from any violent or illegal acts they might involve themselves in.

One of the first things to look at when entrenching your home is points-of-entry. This can be doors or windows around the house that intruders can enter from. Make sure that all exterior doors have a dead bolt lock on them. Chain style locks are good too, but can be torn off much easier. If a pandemic does occur, you may want to add dead bolt locks to inner rooms of your home as well. Check all the windows in your home as too. Make sure they all stay locked. A quick and easy step to increase the security of a window is to drill a hole through the wood casing on one side of the window, where the upper and lower window frames overlap. Once this is done, you can insert a nail or metal pin through the hole, locking the upper and lower window together.

If someone breaks the glass out to unlock the window this will help to prevent them from opening it easily, even if it is unlocked since it would probably take some time for them to figure out why the window will not open. By that point, the intruder would hopefully have made enough noise to alert you to their presence. If you need to get the window opened yourself, simply pull out the pin or nail with a knife, hammer or pliers. If you want to go further with this, you can also look at adding security bars to windows that aren't needed as fire exits, but be careful and leave yourself escape points on opposite ends of your home. Many people die each year thanks in part to being trapped inside their homes by security bars. Consider alternate ways of sealing up all but a few points-of-entry, particularly those on ground level. Sheets of ¾" plywood or even 2x4's covering windows and screwed or nailed to the studs on the inside of the house is a good method that's easily reversed later on. For a sturdier alternative, think about actually bricking-up various windows or doorways. Be sure not to overlook the potential of windows or balconies on an upper floor as possible points-of-entry. A simple ladder could allow intruders to gain entry unexpectedly in upper levels as well. By sealing-up all but a few key entry areas, you maintain control of where intruders can or cannot easily, get into your home. By doing this, you can plan-out entrenchment locations in the likely event of a home invasion.

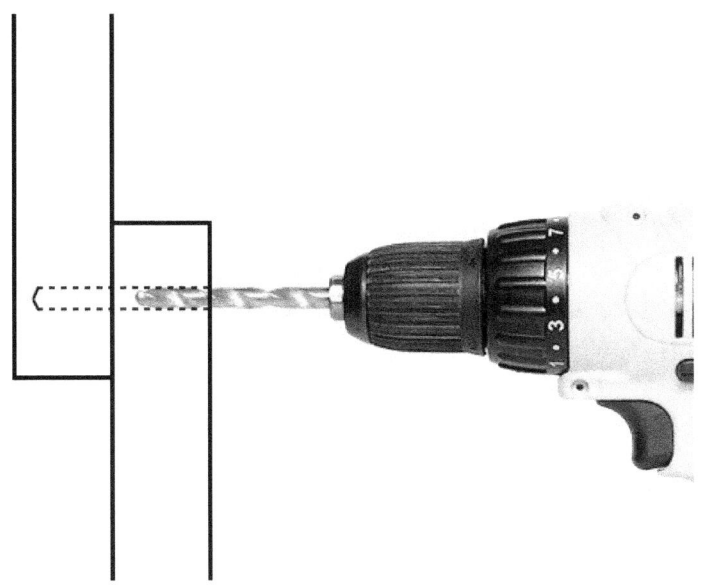

Example of How to Drill Locking Nail Hole through Window Frames

One way of doing this might be to build a make-shift fox hole or turret in your foyer, or upstairs balcony. This can be done by simply filling zip-lock bags with sand and stacking them in a circle, semi-circular or linear formation. The bags of sand will help to protect you in the event of a firefight from

intruders, since the sand can shield the occupants and prevent penetration of most types of rounds. During a pandemic, it would be a good idea to assign shifts to monitor the key point(s) of entry and guard against intruders. Two to four hour shifts are long enough to be effective without running the risk of someone getting overly tired or bored and accidentally falling asleep. Also, if you have three or more people to take shifts, it would allow for a significant amount of down-time for others to sleep, rest, exercise or do whatever to decompress.

If you do not own a gun, now would be a great time to exercise your Constitutional right to bear arms and go buy one. If you are not familiar with guns and the different types of bullet sizes, it's easy to get confused about what to look for. Here are a few tips. Do not fall for the urge to get a small, extremely low-powered gun that shoots .22, .25 or .32 caliber bullets. Smaller caliber handguns tend to jam more easily, and often first-time purchasers will make the mistake of thinking that a smaller gun will be easier to handle and less intimidating to have around the house. However, intimidation is actually half of the equation when selecting the right type of firearm. A gun that looks big and scary will make anyone who sees it think twice before doing something dumb. This does not mean you have to get a huge .44 magnum like Dirty Harry. In fact I would only recommend getting a revolver as a secondary weapon. When selecting a gun, look at what's called "auto cartridge pistols" (Figure 8). These handguns store their bullets in a clip or magazine.

There are two reasons for selecting this type of weapon. First, loading and unloading is quick and easy. With the push of a button the empty clip slides out of the bottom of the handle, and a fully loaded one can take its place. If you want to unload the weapon for storage, all you have to do is remove the clip. Second, the recoil from an auto cartridge pistol is

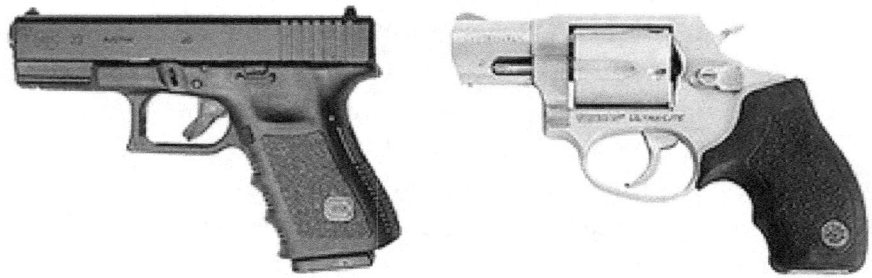

Handgun Types, Pistol (left) and Revolver (right)

typically much less than that of a revolver. This has to do with the sliding chamber which sits on top of the gun. Each time the gun is fired, the gun is designed to utilize the force to slide the chamber back so the expended bullet casing can be ejected and replaced with a new bullet automatically. The resulting action is much like a shock absorber on your car. This means that instead of the gun kicking up into the air every time it's fired and having to reacquire the target again prior to squeezing off another round, you can just continue to aim at the target while discharging rounds.

For women I would recommend a .380 caliber, 9mm or .40 caliber pistol. With the proper ammunition, these will generally have enough stopping power without an enormous amount of flash and recoil.

For men I'd recommend a 10mm, .40 or .45 caliber pistol. The .45 caliber will have the most stopping power and the potential to knock someone to the ground from the shear force of the round. However, the .45 caliber bullet is a subsonic round so penetrating heavier doors or walls would be better

suited for 10mm handguns which are supersonic in nature. The .40 caliber pistol is one of the most popular on the market and is used by roughly 70% of law enforcement in the US.

Whatever caliber pistol you decide to go with, be sure you stock-up on the right type of ammunition as well. A gun without bullets is a useless item. I recommend getting either hollow point bullets, which expand on impact, or Hydra-Shok® which is like a hybrid variant of the hollow point that provides better penetration as well as expansion.

In addition to a handgun, it would be a good idea to have some type of rifle or shot gun on hand as well. A nice pump action 12 gauge shot gun are often the most affordable. They make great defensive weapons, can hold multiple rounds, are simple to load and operate, and can also be used for hunting all kinds of animals and game. Ammunition for shotguns is also extremely flexible and come in sizes from 2¾" shells to 3½". The longer the shell, the more powerful the blast and the further it will go. However, if you use smaller/shorter shells, you can typically fit more rounds into the gun. The shell types come in everything from "birdshot" (dozens of tiny bbs), "buckshot" (a few larger size pellets), to a "slug" (a single solid lead projectile). Most experts agree that buckshot is the best type of defensive ammo when it comes to knocking down and stopping an aggressor. Your aim doesn't have to be very accurate as the pellets quickly disperse into a wide pattern once they leave the barrel. In fact, the shorter the barrel is, the wider the pattern. Look at shotguns with an 18" barrel if possible. This is the shortest barrel allowed by law without a special permit. The three most common variations of buckshot are known as triple ought(000), double ought(00) and No. 4. The 000 contains the largest pellets, the 00 are smaller but more of them, and the No. 4 resembles large bbs. For example, a 3" 000 buckshot shell usually contains 10 large pellets, the 00 contains 15 and the No. 4 contains 41. If your aim isn't horrible, I'd recommend stocking up on 000, but having all three on hand isn't a bad idea either. You could even alternate different types of rounds that you load into the gun.

If you're experienced with rifles and targeting distant object, then the world's your oyster in the rifle department. I would recommend either a .223 or a .308 rifle. Both can be used effectively for hunting & self defense, and both are the weapons of choice by SWAT units around the country; and the ammo for both is readily available. The .223 is a smaller round and will probably save you money when trying to stock up on ammo. The .308 is larger and has more penetrating power. Either round is capable of passing through a medium size tree trunk at close range, which means that both will penetrate doors and walls as well; so if you have neighbors or live in a neighborhood where you're surrounded by other houses, these weapons should be reserved for use outdoors or in areas of the home that are surrounded by brick and/or concrete, such as a basement.

Remember, you must secure and defend your property and resources for the survival of you and your family. Post signs on the doors and/or windows of your home to warn potential intruders to stay away. Anybody wandering by looking for a house to loot is more likely to break into one that is either unoccupied or occupied by residents who are unprepared or unable to defend themselves. Stay alert and always be on guard. In desperate times people can become irrational and unruly, with total disregard for the law or even other people's lives.

Medical Supplies

Right now the most important medical item to purchase is the antiviral drug known as Tamiflu® (oseltamivir). This is the only type of medicine on the market today which is capable of combating the infectious virus, although no one knows for

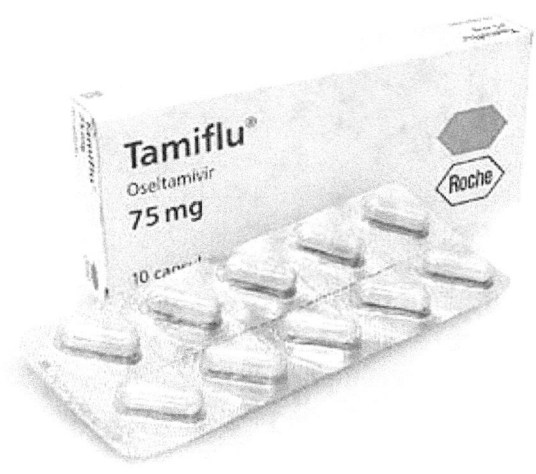

Tamiflu® Antiviral Dose Pack by Roche

certain just how effective it would be against the H5N1 strain. It comes in a dose pack of 10 capsules. At the first sign of infection, the victim must start taking the capsules twice a day, once in the morning and once at night, through completion. If treatment is delayed, there is a good chance that it won't even work. Remember, antivirals such as Tamiflu® will only halt the advancement of the illness. They will not provide any lasting immunization to the virus. Therefore, even if someone takes the medicine and recovers, re-infection is still possible. The capsules should be stored at room temperature below 77°F (25°C) and kept in a dry place. Be sure to get at least one dose pack for every member of your family.

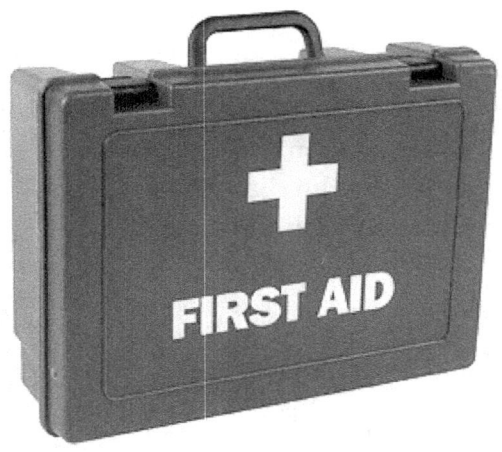

Standard First Aid Kit

Having a first-aid kit on hand is another great idea, but besides the obvious first-aid items, such as band-aids, hydrogen peroxide, alcohol, antibiotic ointment and gauze wrap, you should also include over-the-counter medications like cough medicine, throat lozenges, aspirin, ibuprofen, naproxen, antacids, antidiarrheals, antihistamines and any prescription medications you are currently on or uses from time to time, such as inhalers. If you have antibiotics to add to your medical supplies it may prove to be invaluable. Just having some of these simple items on hand could head-off a potentially more serious medical problem that might need professional attention later on.

Fuels

When preparing to hunker down long-term, it's easy to forget what you might need to store in case you have to get out of Dodge, i.e. - gasoline. Look at storing enough gas to fill you car's tank up at least once. If a pandemic starts, try to top-off what ever is in your gas tank. When storing gasoline, there are a few things you must remember. First, never store gas cans without their approved cap or lid. Second, never store them where they could accidentally be knocked over and spilled. Third, never store them near a water heater, heat source or any type of open flame. You do not want any section of your home going up in flames, especially if the fire department is not coming. Fourth, never store gasoline inside your home. Fumes and vapors from evaporating gasoline not only creates long-term health risks, but they can also cause nausea, dizziness and even death. Finally, when storing gasoline for any length of time, you must add fuel stabilizer to keep it fresh. Without fuel stabilizer mixed in with the gas, it will lose its ability to perform properly. Trying to run it through your car's engine would result in gummy varnish-like film and residue which can clog up fuel lines, carburetors and fuel injectors, essentially destroying your engine. One thing to do in order to avoid wasting fuel stabilizer & gasoline is to periodically use each can in a sequenced rotation. When your car gets half empty, pour one of the cans into the tank. When it's time to refill the car, take that can with you to the gas station and refill it. If you practice this type of rotation with your stored fuel, you should not need to add fuel stabilizer to any of the cans until a pandemic occurs.

Another fuel source to consider storing is propane. Propane is bought and stored in a liquid form called liquid propane gas(LPG) and thus more fuel energy can be stored in a relatively smaller space. Compressed natural gas(CNG), largely methane, is another gas used as fuel but requires very high pressure to liquefy. Because of this, CNG is less efficient to store due to the larger tank volume required. There are many uses for propane as a back-up fuel source. In addition to propane heaters and stoves, some companies actually have propane powered refrigerators as well, which are said to be

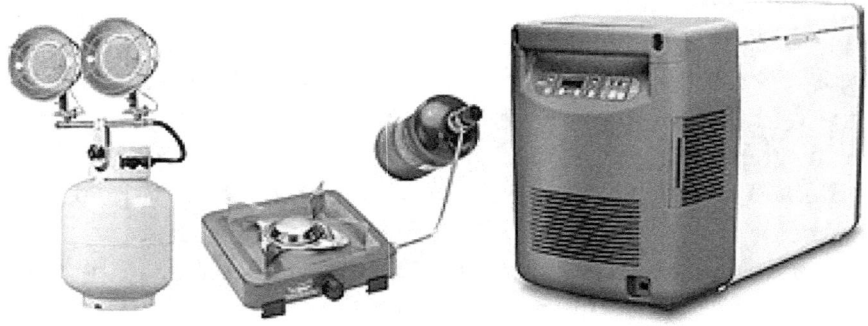

Some Examples of Various Propane Powered Devices
Space Heater (left), Stove (center) & Refrigerator (right)

extremely efficient. Propane tanks come in an array of shapes and sizes to fit practically any need; everything from small handheld bottles to huge horizontal storage tanks that can be mounted behind your house or shed.

Other Items

One way to look at preparing for a pandemic is to imagine what you would want and need if you were going to an extremely remote area of the world for an extended period of time. Think of what you would take to occupy yourself and companions. Items you might not see for several months or even years. Things or activities that could make your life easier and more enjoyable, or counter act boredom, as well as things that could be used for bartering. Here is a brief list of items which I would suggest:

- Stationary, Journals & Writing Instruments
- Sketch Pads, Pencils & Paints
- Coloring Books & Crayons
- Board Games/Card Games
- Books and Novels
- Extra Batteries
- CD or MP3 Players
- Portable Radio or TV
- DVD's & Portable DVD Player
- Handheld Electronic Games
- Cellular Phones
- Phone Numbers & Addresses of Family/Friends
- Matches & Lighters
- Propane Camping Stove
- Propane or Kerosene Heaters
- Gasoline, Kerosene, Propane, Charcoal
- Fire Extinguisher
- Extra Clothing, Underwear, Boots & Coveralls
- Sponges, Washcloths & Towels
- Emergency Blankets & Inflatable Mattresses
- Duct Tape
- Rope and/or Nylon String
- Trash Bags
- Household Cleaning Supplies
- Unopened Toys & Presents
- Musical Instruments
- Potting Soil & Seeds
- Telescope and/or Binoculars
- Cash & Change ($200 Minimum)
- Gold & Silver Bars and/or Coins

Chapter 4
Surviving the Aftermath

If you have ever wondered what would happen when news breaks of a bird flu outbreak in the US, just think back to what generally happens when there's an announcement of a snow storm or hurricane. I have seen it first hand. People rush out to the grocery store and buy up all the milk and bread first, followed by sodas, snacks, canned goods, batteries, etc. - and that is just for a small snow flurry. Once an announcement has been made of a contagion like H5N1 hitting the country, panic stricken people will be scrambling to purchase everything imaginable to help them survive. Grocery stores would most certainly be cleaned out in less than twenty-four (24) hours. The first ones to the stores would most likely horde all they could get into their cars, and max out their credit card to do so. Everyone with a spare gas can would be emptying what was left at their local gas stations. Pandemonium and fear would most certainly grip those who were totally unprepared to deal with such sudden shortages and chaotic events like fights at the checkout counters, riots in the streets and the almost instantaneous devaluing of the US dollar. Once products disappear from store shelves, money will become practically worthless compared to the value of a can of soup or a box of rice. Anyone expecting FEMA or the federal government to come to their immediate rescue should take a good hard look at the victims of hurricane Katrina, and how long it took just to get food and supplies to those people. If you had to supply the entire nation as opposed to a state or two, you quickly get a glimpse of just how big this problem is going to be. With the usual supply lines dwindling, truck drivers either sick or unwilling to take the risks, long-term shortages of everyday items and amenities would be sure to follow. Any truckers that did make it from depots to their destinations may find themselves quickly overwhelmed by armed attackers in search of food and supplies for themselves or their families.

Those who would be desperate enough to venture out would be putting themselves and their families at risk of contracting and further spreading the virus.

As earlier stated, your greatest chance of surviving an ensuing pandemic would be to stay indoors and isolate you and your loved ones from outside visitors as much as possible. Venturing outside or making the mistake of letting others into your home could jeopardize the health and lives of everyone inside. Do not do it. The World Health Organization predicts that it will take a minimum of six (6) months or more for a vaccine to be made available to the public after a bird flu pandemic has begun, so isolating your family from outside contact until everyone is vaccinated would be imperative.

If you have children, you should plan on home schooling them. Local schools are sure to be one of the first institutions to be shut down during a global pandemic. Experts predict that schools would be closed for a year or more. At the height of a pandemic, with funeral homes and cemeteries overwhelmed, schools would most likely be used as morgues to house the dead. Keep several educational workbooks on hand. They are inexpensive and can be readily found at your local book store.

With many people infected and many others dying of starvation, exposure, violence, etc., it will be critical to your mental health to find ways of distracting yourself and your family from the ensuing chaos. Plan some fun daily activities to pass the time. Board games and card games can be good way to interact with each other. Books and novels can not only educate and entertain the mind, but can consume countless hours of free time as well. One book I would recommend having on your shelf is an atlas of the area you live in. If for any reason you need to evacuate or move away from the area, an atlas could be your road map to salvation. In addition to highways, roads and bridges, an atlas can point you to other places of interest, such as lakes, rivers and streams, caves, fallout shelters, military bases, airports and landing strips, etc.

Defense Strategy

In order to improve your survival skills in the midst of a bird flu pandemic, you will have to change the way you perceive your immediate surroundings, your friends and neighbors and your world in general. As difficult as it would be to isolate yourself and family from outside contact, it will be unimaginably difficult to contend with the cries and pleas of those who may beg you for food or supplies. After all, you would not be human if you did not feel some kind of sympathy or remorse for friends, neighbors or unfortunate strangers who may be dying of infection, starvation, dehydration or exposure, right outside your home. How you choose to deal with these situations if they arise, will not only serve to define you as a person, but could also determine whether or not you and your family survive. So put some forethought into various scenarios and discuss them with your family and/or spouse before such circumstances arise so that your decisions will be well planned, not rushed or made in haste. I have often wondered what I would do if my son's little friends and their families in our neighborhood were on the verge of starvation or in desperate need of supplies. One thing to remember is that you cannot supply everyone with food and provisions unless you are really wealthy and have stored enough away to hand out to all those who come by asking. The downside to being generous can easily be seen when you look at how juvenile gangs behave in impoverished countries. They will usually find an unsuspecting tourist who is well off, like an American. Then they will beg them for money, food, candy, anything they can get. When the tourist stops to pull out their wallet or give them something, they are instantly overwhelmed and taken for everything they have. I have no reason to believe that this same type of thinking would become common place here during such an event.

Making Alliances

In the wake of such a pandemic event, it might be wise to establish alliances with local friends and neighbors. There is always strength in numbers. A rogue gang of thieves or hoodlums will think twice about intruding on a tight-knit community or neighborhood rather than one that is in disarray. Keeping an eye out for each other is a first step back to law, order and normalcy.

Food and Supplies

We have already discussed food and various supplies in the Advanced Preparations section, but what about supplies that you might need in the aftermath of a worldwide pandemic. What kind of supplies and food stores will you need for ultra-long-term situations that may extend beyond a six (6) month period? One thing to consider might be a few simple yard tools such as shovels, rakes, hoes, etc. If you find that you need to grow your own food in order to supplement your dwindling food stores, these could prove invaluable. A few bulk bags of non-hybrid seed to plant may prove to be a real life saver down the road as well. Obviously what you can successfully grow will depend on your location and ecological conditions. Check what types of fruits and/or vegetables thrive in your area and consider stocking seeds for those particular plants. I like the idea of also planting vegetation which may require little if any interaction, such as melons or plants that grow on vines. These could include watermelons, cantaloupes, squash, pumpkins, etc. Plants that grow primarily underground may be easier to culture and keep longer as well. These might include potatoes, peanuts, carrots, etc. Again, do a little research to determine what would grow best in your region throughout the year.

Monetary Alternatives

If you have enough extra monetary resources at your disposal, I would recommend storing up on gold or silver bullion bars and/or coins. If cash becomes devalued or more than likely obsolete, precious metals would most likely become the replacement currency in just about every country or region affected. Focus on getting lots of small bars(ingots) or coins rather than just a few large ones. Silver dollars, quarters and dimes dated before 1965 contain 90% silver. Since they are so plentiful at pawn shops and online auctions, they are ideal for bartering or purchasing. As far as gold goes, one gram, five gram and five gram ingots should be suitable for trade.

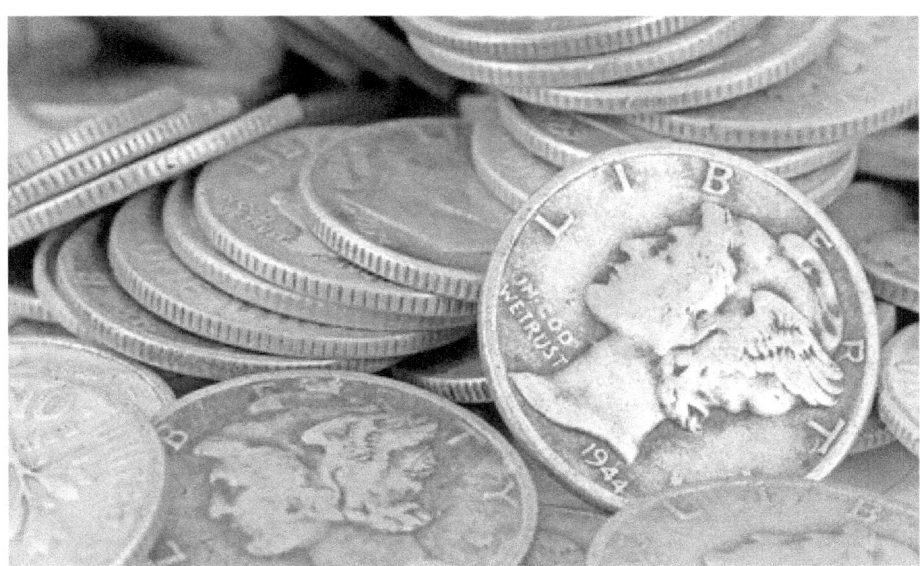

Example of a Pre-1965 US Coins which Contain 90% Silver

Food Banks & Soup Kitchens

Ultimately the government or other relief organizations may try to reestablish food chains to the populous via food banks or soup kitchens. This would be terrific if a vaccination for the H5N1 strain has been developed and administered to you and your family by then, a potentially deadly visit if it has not. Make sure that you and your family have been inoculated before risking exposure to such a congested public venue. If you are able, take your firearms with you for continued protection. In a post apocalyptic event such as the bird flu pandemic, there may be many survivors who may try to take advantage of a strained or non-existent law enforcement, so stay aware of your surroundings if you have to venture out.

Chapter 5
Surviving the Wait

Six months to a year is an awful long time to be boxed-up in your house, isolated from friends, relatives and your surrounding community. Words like "stir-crazy" and "cabin fever" come to mind. Obviously you and your family, particularly those with children, will have to come up with creative ways to keep yourselves preoccupied. Board games

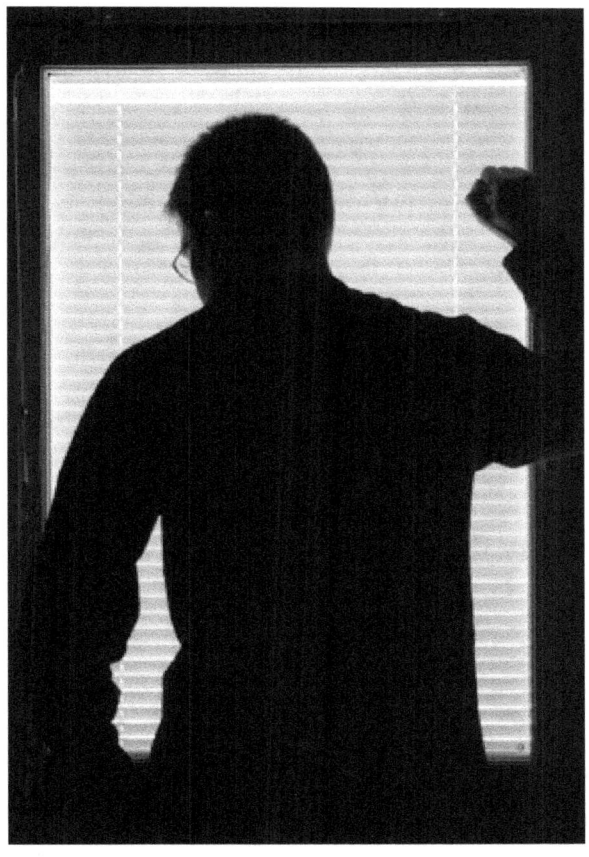

Waiting for the Pandemic to End

and strategy games work well as they allow you to use your mind and typically involve more than just 2 people. A good game of Monopoly$_{TM}$ can last for several hours and easily involve 4-6 players. Other games to consider are chess, checkers, card games, etc. Some of my personal favorites are Uno$_{TM}$, Skipbo$_{TM}$, and Rook$_{TM}$.

Hobbies are one of the best ways to entertain your self while creating useful and/or decorative items since they directly involve you and are associated with your personal interests. Consider activities such as writing, sketching, painting, knitting, sewing, pottery, sculpting, whittling, model building, etc. Items you create could serve as birthday, Christmas or anniversary gifts. In addition, some of these items may be useful later on for bartering with others.

Other activities could be geared toward excising together. These activities might include such things as arm wrestling, throwing a ball or Frisbee, fencing, Tai Chi, Yoga, aerobics, dancing, weight lifting, fencing, etc. Exercising will also help to improve your defensive abilities and keep your immune system functioning at its peak level.

Exercise the brain. Play games like charades, tic-tac-toe or hangman. Keep a dictionary on hand and have a spelling bee. If you have a map or globe, see who can find a particular island or country the quickest. Tell stories. A well told story, fiction or nonfiction, can invoke mental imagery and be a great alternative to television.

Escape from reality by reading a book. Nothing relaxes the mind better than a good novel or short story. Be sure to stock-up on classics as well as other books with topics that are of interest to you and your family. A stack of old magazines could serve as a fun way to give your kids something to look forward to by letting them have a different issue each week.

Above all, be creative with the activities you come up with and have fun doing them. It is good to have planned events but being spontaneous and spur of the moment will go a long way in breaking-up the monotony as well.

Keeping Your Sanity

The resulting horrific events that a bird flu pandemic might produce may prove to be very desensitizing to the human psyche. Seeing people dying in the streets unattended or bodies of dead people lining the sidewalks could be enough to push any normal person over the edge. The death of friends and loved ones can churn-up emotions of grief and despair and coping with such losses will be paramount. Add a devastated economy, global unrest, interrupted utilities and basic services and the uncertainty of a better tomorrow, and the strain can become unbearably depressing. In times like these, you will need to constantly encourage each other. Be there for your family and talk about how you feel and items of

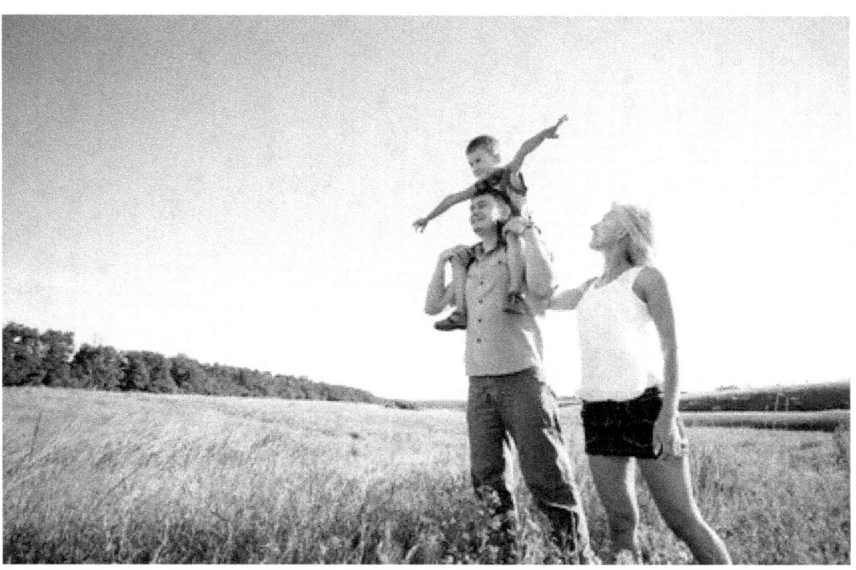

Family Spending Time Together

concern. Reassure your family and discus what is going on and how you can deal with certain issues together. Rely on your faith for comfort and guidance. Keep separated loved ones in your thoughts and prayers. If a dyer situation arises, try not to burden your children with the unnecessary details. Stay strong for your family. The last thing your children need is to see mommy or daddy having a psychotic break. Most of all, love on each other and help each other keep it together mentally, emotionally and spiritually.

No normal person likes to entertain the thoughts of what a pandemic caused by the H5N1 virus would produce; the unimaginable consequences and tolls on our families, nation and world. All too often we tend to quickly shelve such ideas in a mental broom closet to keep us from having to deal with difficult or negative ideas. The reality of this situation is this; the contagion H5N1 bird flu virus does exist, right now, somewhere on the planet today! It is just a matter of time before the virus mutates to the point that it is able to jump species and infect humans unchecked. There is currently no vaccine to protect us from an outbreak and it will take six (6) to twelve (12) months for one to be developed and distributed once the virus has begun to spread.

Hopefully after reading this book, you will have gained some useful insight toward preparation and safeguards against an H5N1 pandemic. In case you're wondering what other people around the country think or know about the avian flu, take a look at the survey that I conducted below. The results may surprise you.

The following survey was conducted online and involved 100 people all across the continental US, including Hawaii. Here are the questions and results:

- ONLINE AVIAN BIRD FLU QUESTIONAIRE -

Have you ever heard of "H5N1"?
Yes 25%
No 74%

Do you know the primary differences between the bird flu and other types of influenza viruses?

Yes 27%

No 73%

Do you think that the bird flu virus is more dangerous or less dangerous than other types of infections such as a common cold, the stomach flu or other types of viruses/infections?

More Dangerous... 55%

Less Dangerous 5%

About the Same 15%

No Idea 25%

Have you ever heard of the H1N1 flu pandemic of 1918?

Yes 36%

No 64%

Do you think the H5N1 bird flu virus is more dangerous or less dangerous than the H1N1 flu virus of 1918?

More Dangerous... 12%

Less Dangerous 8%

About the Same 16%

No Idea 64%

If you heard on the news tomorrow that a bird flu pandemic had spread to the US how would you feel?

Wouldn't Be Concerned 9%

Would Be Mildly Concerned............................. 46%

Would Be Very Concerned 38%

Would Be Panic Stricken..................................... 6%

Do you believe that the C.D.C. (Center for Disease Control) or W.H.O. (World Health Organization) have already developed a cure for the H5N1 bird flu virus?

Yes 12%

No 55%

No Idea 34%

About how long do you think it would take the US government to get a bird flu vaccine to people around the country if a pandemic did occur?
1 Week or Less 2%
2 to 4 Weeks 11%
1 to 2 Months 13%
2 to 4 Months 5%
4 to 6 Months 10%
6 to 8 Months 6%
8 to 10 Months 3%
10 Months to a Year 31%
No Idea 20%

What all would you do if you heard that this same virus was killing 6 out of 10 people who contracted it? (Check all that Apply)
Warn Family, Friends & Neighbors 75%
Stock Up on Food, Water & Supplies............................... 51%
Pray and/or Seek Out Spiritual Guidance...................... 46%
Go to Doctor and Get a Flu Shot..................................... 41%
Buy Gloves & Face Masks... 38%
Start Taking Lots of Vitamin C 35%
Plan to Stay Indoors Until it was Over 35%
Buy Weapons & Ammunition... 12%
Move to Avoid Human Contact 10%
Cash Out Stocks, Bonds, Etc. 9%
Leave the Country Altogether... 7%
Invest in Precious Metals to Barter With 5%
Quit Your Job and/or Change Careers............................. 4%
Leave Your House/Declare Bankruptcy 1%

How long do you think it would take for such a pandemic to come to an end?
1 to 3 Months 4%
3 to 6 Months 9%

6 to 9 Months 11%
9 to 12 Months 7%
1 Year or More 38%
No Idea 32%

If you, a family member or loved one contracted this illness and a treatment was available which might improve their odds of survival, what is the maximum amount of money would you consider to be fair for this treatment if the quantities to the public were extremely limited?
It Should be Free 50%
$100-$500 .... 17%
$500-$1,000 .... 6%
$1,000-$2,500 .... 0%
$2,500-$5,000 .... 4%
$5,000-$10,000 .... 2%
Any Amount 21%

Do you have food, water and/or supplies specifically stored up for such an event?
Yes 29%
No 71%

If so, how long do you think you and your dependants could survive on what you have stored up?
1 Week or Less 51%
1 Month or Less 27%
2 Months or Less 7%
3 Months or Less 5%
4 Months or Less 2%
5 Months or Less 0%
6 Months or Less 3%
6 Months or More 5%

If a friend, neighbor or coworker came to your home during a pandemic and they appeared to be okay, but you weren't sure if they were infected or not, would you let them in?

Yes 25%
No 29%
Not Sure 46%

If relatives came to your home during a pandemic and they appeared to be okay, but again, you weren't sure if they were infected or not, would you let them in?
Yes 55%
No 13%
Not Sure 32%

Do you have any weapons or firearms to defend yourself and/or your family (not including kitchen knives, gardening tools or sporting equipment)?
Yes 36%
No 64%

Do you and your family have a planned out evacuation strategy in the even that you must suddenly leave the area or seek shelter during an emergency?
Yes 28%
No 72%

If a global pandemic such as this did occur, how would you survive financially?
Continue to working regardless of the risks 23%
Work from home through your own business 11%
Live on social security, retirement or 401k 5%
Receive charity from family or friends 3%
Independent means or savings 16%
No Idea 42%

Here are some of the comments that people posted after taking the survey...

-- ONLINE AVIAN BIRD FLU COMMENTS --

"I imagine chaos and anarchy would very quickly seize the American population, I'd just try to stay below the radar. If I were to get infected, I'd most likely rely on past health to pull me through."

"I would take precautions, but life goes on. I live across country from my family. I would probably get home to them and we would figure out what to do from there."

"I consider myself seventy-five percent healthier than ANYONE I know, yet I am fearful of an accident removing my independence. Three of my sisters depend on me emotionally and financially."

"In a novel which speculates that we would be thrown into anarchy from such a pandemic, in my opinion there would have to be a massive percentages of deaths (over 50% total population) or an opportunistic invasion from another country. The bird flu alone isn't likely to create the hysteria required for anarchy to occur."

"Interesting questions. I am prepared for an earthquake with food, water, generator, gas and weapons. I could use it for this but the plan would be different."

"I suspect that this so-called bird flu is a bit of a hoax. It's a manufactured panic used to gain a greater degree of control over the population. People in China get sick because they're walking around bare footed in chicken coops."

"Very thought provoking survey."

"This is a terrifying scenario that I would never want to be a part of. Nor would I want to hear of anyone anywhere dealing with such a horrid epidemic."

"Could this happen for real?"

"This was a bit of an eye opener."

"Okay, so I know its coming; I'm completely unprepared and so is my government. I have no money to stockpile anything or to live off of for that matter should commodities even be available. I certainly don't expect that a foreign country would let me in, in the event of an outbreak in the US."

"It sounds like you are talking about this as if its 28 days later... way to scare the crap out of me."

"Considering the constant flow of visitors to my home state (Hawaii), if this virus were to go pandemic on the US mainland, Japan or Australia, we would be involved very quickly. Since the other ongoing hazards here (volcano, hurricane, earthquake, etc) are a constant threat, I consider myself fairly well prepared with food stocks, medical supplies, and advanced training. However, the reality of a worldwide pandemic could go much deeper than the threats of local disasters."

"Even with no money I would still attempt to live somewhere I could grow my own food, collect rain water and stay remote."

Appendix
Helpful Links and Suppliers

American Safe Room
This company specializes in the design and installation of safe rooms and filtration systems.
www.americansaferoom.com

British Broadcast Corporation (BBC)
They are based in England and cover global news and events.
www.bbc.co.uk

Center for Disease Control (CDC)
The CDC is based in Atlanta, GA, and is a government run institution responsible for evaluating and responding to any type of viral outbreaks or pandemics which may pose a threat to the United States.
www.cdc.gov

Euro Health Pharmacy
This pharmacy is based in the UK and sells hard-to-find medicine and antiviral drugs online.
www.eurohealthpharmacy.com

Flu Facts
This is an informative website maintained by Roche Laboratories, which contains write-ups to address flu symptoms, treatments and resources.
www.flufacts.com

Genius Goods
This company offers several models of refrigerators that can not only run on electricity, but propane as well.
www.propanerefrigerator.us

Pandemic Flu
This is an official government website managed by the U.S. Department of Health & Human Services. It contains information on the most recent flu related events.
www.pandemicflu.gov

MRE Star
MRE Star is a company that offers Meals Ready to Eat (MRE's), that are prepackaged and made for long-term storage. Most can retain their freshness and last for years on the shelf. Meals can even be purchased with individual flameless heaters to warm the food.
www.mrestar.com

Roche Pharmaceuticals
This is the company which manufactures Tamiflu®, an antiviral treatment designed to combat the onset of a flu virus after exposure.
www.rocheusa.com

Wikipedia
Wikipedia is a free, multilingual encyclopedia project supported by the non-profit Wikimedia Foundation. Information about the H5N1 and other viruses can be researched here in detail.
www.wikipedia.org

World Health Organization (WHO)
WHO is the directing and coordinating authority for providing leadership on global health matters for the United Nations(UN). The organization provides technical support to various countries and monitors and assesses health trends worldwide.
www.who.int

About the Author

Victor Chase graduated with a Bachelors degree in Computer Science. He spent over 20 years working in the defense contracting industry, where he was granted a secret level security clearance from the Department of Defense and served for several years as a senior research analyst prior to becoming the general manager for a defense firm.

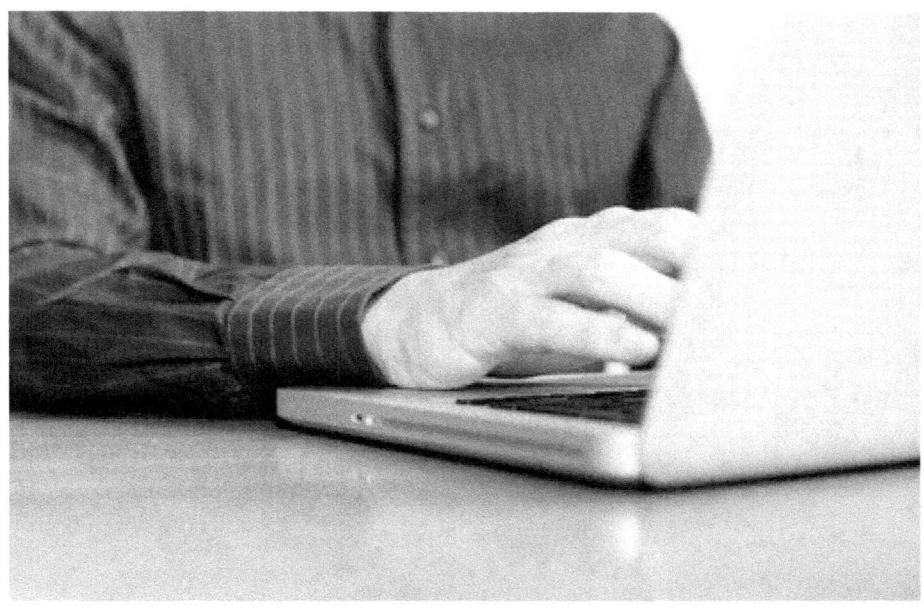

Victor Hard at Work on His Next Literary Compilation

Since the start of his career, Mr. Chase has worked with several aerospace companies, and governmental entities such as the Department of Education, Homeland Security and the Central Intelligence Agency. His involvement has directly contributed to the successful outcome of many projects and operations.

Today he continues to live in the Southeast, where he enjoys spending time with his young son and taking trips to the beach in his spare time.